The Amazing Mediterranean Meat Cookbook

A Complete Collection of Meat Recipes to Start Your Mediterranean Diet and Boost Your Taste

Raymond Morton

Table of contents

Parsley Pork and Rice

Prep time: 10 minutes I **Cooking time:** 40 minutes I
Servings: 4

Ingredients:

- 1 pound pork stew meat, cubed
- 2 tablespoons avocado oil
- 1 yellow onion, chopped
- 1 cup brown rice
- 3 cups vegetable stock
- 2 teaspoons sweet paprika
- 1 teaspoon fennel seeds, crushed
- A pinch of salt and black pepper
- 1 tablespoon parsley, chopped

Directions:

1. Heat up a pan with the oil over medium-high heat, add the onion and the meat and brown for 10 minutes.

2. Add the rest of the ingredients, toss, cook over medium heat for 30 minutes more, divide between plates and serve.

Nutrition info per serving: calories 440, fat 13.9, fiber 3.2, carbs 40.6, protein 37.4

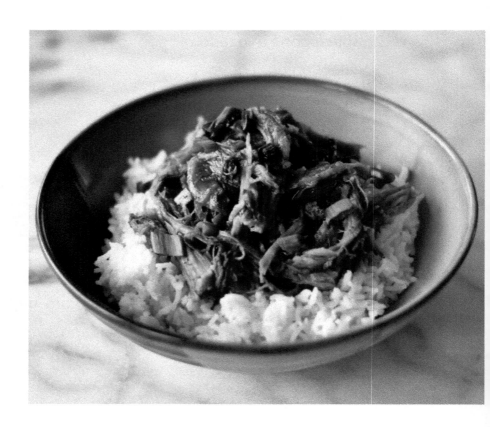

Dill Pork

Prep time: 10 minutes I **Cooking time:** 45 minutes I
Servings: 4

Ingredients:

- 2 pounds pork meat, cubed
- 1 yellow onion, chopped
- 2 tablespoons olive oil
- 1 cup vegetable stock
- 1 teaspoon caraway seeds
- A pinch of salt and black pepper
- 2 tablespoons dill, chopped

Directions:

1. Heat up a pan with the oil over medium heat, add the onion and sauté for 5 minutes.
2. Add the meat and brown for 5 minutes more.
3. Add the rest of the ingredients, toss, cook over medium heat for 35 minutes, divide between plates sand serve.

Nutrition info per serving: calories 300, fat 12.8, fiber 6, carbs 12, protein 16

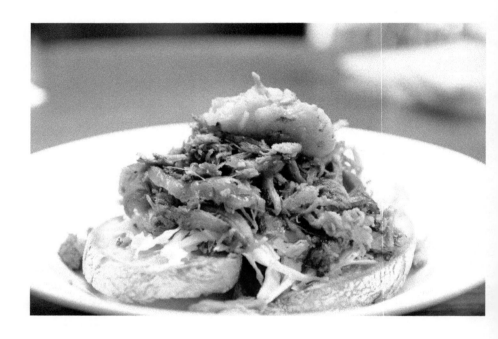

Pork with Peas

Prep time: 10 minutes I **Cooking time:** 40 minutes I

Servings: 4

Ingredients:

- 2 pounds pork stew meat, cut into strips
- ½ cup corn
- ½ cup green peas
- 2 tablespoons olive oil
- ½ cup yellow onion, chopped
- 3 tablespoons coconut aminos
- ½ cup vegetable stock
- A pinch of salt and black pepper

Directions:

1. Heat up a pan with the oil over medium heat, add the meat and the onion and brown for 10 minutes.
2. Add the corn and the other ingredients, toss, cook over medium heat for 30 minutes more, divide between plates and serve.

Nutrition info per serving: calories 250, fat 4, fiber 6, carbs 9.7, protein 12

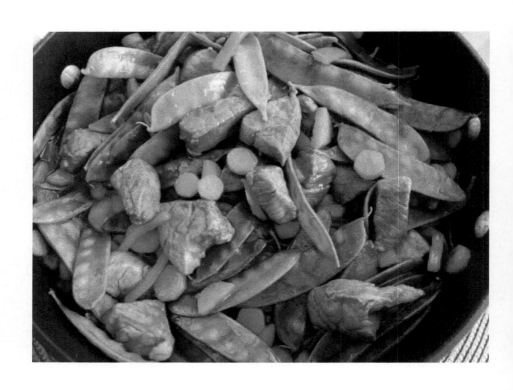

Smoked Pork with Carrots

Prep time: 10 minutes I **Cooking time:** 1 hour I
Servings: 4

Ingredients:

- 1 pound pork meat, cubed
- 2 carrots, sliced
- 2 tablespoons avocado oil
- 1 yellow onion, chopped
- A pinch of salt and black pepper
- ¼ teaspoon smoked paprika
- ½ cup tomato sauce

Directions:

1. Heat up a pan with the oil over medium-high heat, add the onion and the meat and brown for 10 minutes.
2. Add the rest of the ingredients, toss, put the pan in the oven and bake at 390 degrees F for 50 minutes.
3. Divide everything between plates and serve.

Nutrition info per serving: calories 300, fat 7, fiber 6, carbs 12, protein 20

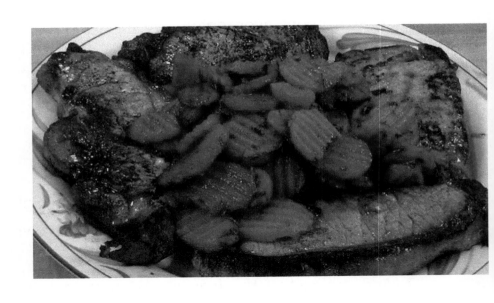

Coconut Pork and Leeks

Prep time: 10 minutes I **Cooking time:** 55 minutes I
Servings: 4

Ingredients:

- 2 pounds pork stew meat, cubed
- 3 leeks, sliced
- 2 tablespoons olive oil
- 1 teaspoon black peppercorns
- 1 tablespoon parsley, chopped
- 2 cups coconut cream
- 1 teaspoon rosemary, dried
- A pinch of salt and black pepper

Directions:

1. Heat up a pan with the oil over medium heat, add the leeks and the meat and brown for 5 minutes.
2. Add the rest of the ingredients, toss, put the pan in the oven and bake at 390 degrees F for 50 minutes.
3. Divide everything into bowls and serve.

Nutrition info per serving: calories 280, fat 5, fiber 7, carbs 12, protein 18

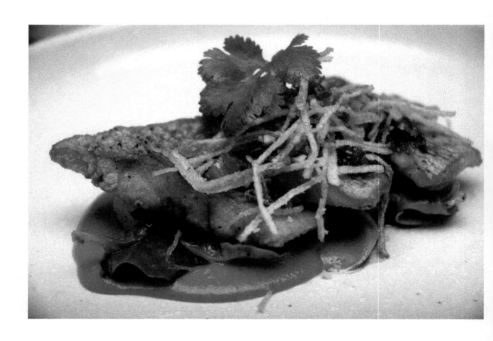

Tarragon Roast

Prep time: 10 minutes I **Cooking time:** 1 hour I

Servings: 4

Ingredients:

- 2 pounds pork loin roast, sliced
- 1 tablespoon tarragon, chopped
- A pinch of salt and black pepper
- 4 garlic cloves, chopped
- 1 teaspoon red pepper, crushed
- ¼ cup olive oil

Directions:

1. In a roasting pan, combine the roast with the tarragon and the other ingredients, toss and bake at 390 degrees F for 1 hour.
2. Divide the mix between plates and serve.

Nutrition info per serving: calories 281, fat 5, fiber 7, carbs 8, protein 10

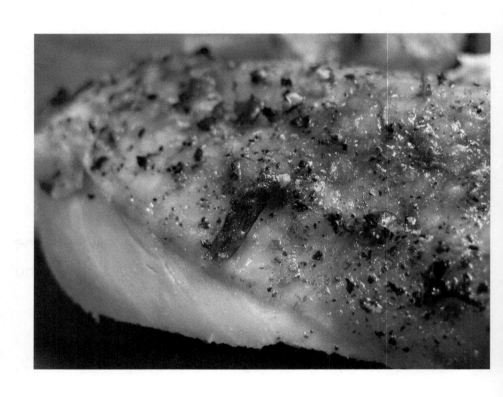

Pork and Onions

Prep time: 10 minutes I **Cooking time:** 1 hour I

Servings: 4

Ingredients:

- 2 pounds pork roast, sliced
- 2 sweet potatoes, peeled and sliced
- 2 tablespoons olive oil
- 1 teaspoon rosemary, dried
- 1 teaspoon turmeric powder
- 2 yellow onions, sliced
- ½ cup veggie stock
- A pinch of salt and black pepper

Directions:

1. In a roasting pan, combine the pork slices with the sweet potatoes, the onions and the other ingredients, toss and bake at 400 degrees F for 1 hours.
2. Divide everything between plates and serve.

Nutrition info per serving: calories 290, fat 4, fiber 7, carbs 10, protein 17

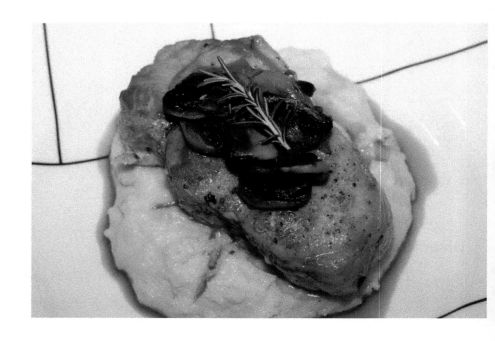

Pork with Pineapple

Prep time: 10 minutes I **Cooking time:** 40 minutes I
Servings: 4

Ingredients:

- 4 pork chops
- 2 tablespoons olive oil
- ½ cup vegetable stock
- 4 scallions, chopped
- 1 cup pineapple, peeled and cubed
- 1 mango, peeled and cubed
- 4 tablespoons lime juice
- 1 handful basil, chopped
- A pinch of salt and cayenne pepper

Directions:

1. Heat up a pan with the oil over medium heat, add the scallions and the meat and brown for 5 minutes.
2. Add the pineapple and the other ingredients, toss, cook over medium heat for 35 minutes more, divide between plates and serve.

Nutrition info per serving: calories 250, fat 5, fiber 6, carbs 8, protein 17

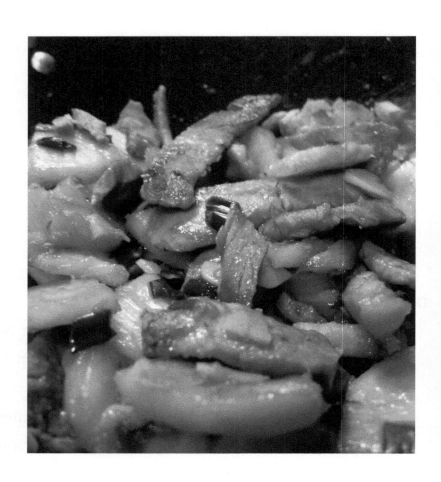

Pork with Celery Mix

Prep time: 10 minutes I **Cooking time:** 40 minutes I

Servings: 4

Ingredients:

- 2 pounds pork stew meat, roughly cubed
- 2 tablespoons olive oil
- 2 tablespoons lemon juice
- 5 garlic cloves, minced
- 2 stalks celery, chopped
- 1 cup Brussels sprouts, trimmed and halved
- A pinch of salt and black pepper
- ½ teaspoon cinnamon powder
- 2 tablespoons parsley, chopped

Directions:

1. Heat up a pan with the oil over medium-high heat, add the garlic and the meat and brown for 5 minutes.
2. Add the celery and the other ingredients, toss, introduce the pan in the oven and cook at 400 degrees F for 35 minutes more.
3. Divide the mix between plates and serve.

Nutrition info per serving: calories 284, fat 4, fiber 4, carbs 9, protein 15

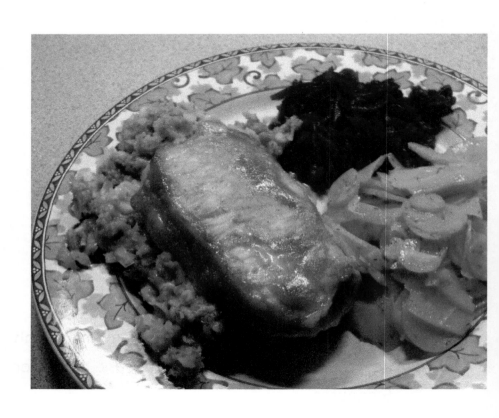

Pork and Green Beans

Prep time: 10 minutes I **Cooking time:** 40 minutes I

Servings: 4

Ingredients:

- 2 pounds pork stew meat, cubed
- 2 tablespoons avocado oil
- ½ cup green beans, trimmed and halved
- 2 tablespoons lime juice
- 1 cup coconut milk
- 1 tablespoon rosemary, chopped
- A pinch of salt and black pepper

Directions:

1. Heat up a pan with the oil over medium heat, add the meat and brown for 5 minutes.
2. Add the rest of the ingredients, toss gently, bring to a simmer and cook over medium heat for 35 minutes more.
3. Divide the mix between plates and serve.

Nutrition info per serving: calories 260, fat 5, fiber 8, carbs 9, protein 13

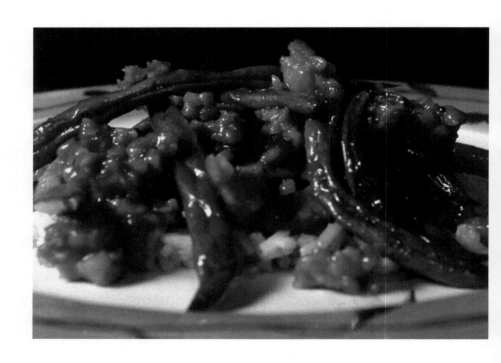

Coconut Lemongrass Pork

Prep time: 10 minutes I **Cooking time:** 30 minutes I

Servings: 4

Ingredients:

- 4 pork chops
- 2 tablespoons olive oil
- 2 spring onions, chopped
- A pinch of salt and black pepper
- ½ cup vegetable stock
- 1 stalk lemongrass, chopped
- 2 tablespoons coconut aminos
- 2 tablespoons cilantro, chopped

Directions:

1. Heat up a pan with the oil over medium-high heat, add the spring onions and the meat and brown for 5 minutes.
2. Add the rest of the ingredients, toss, and cook everything over medium heat for 25 minutes more.
3. Divide the mix between plates and serve.

Nutrition info per serving: calories 290, fat 4, fiber 6, carbs 8, protein 14

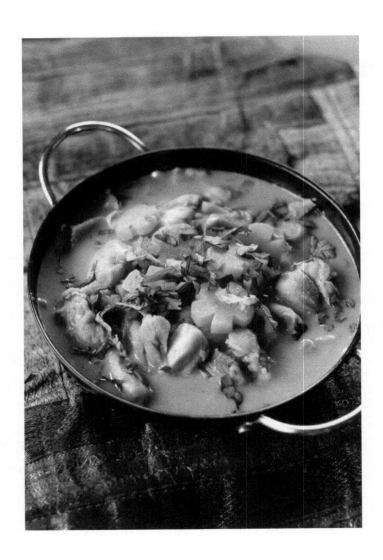

Balsamic Pork with Olives

Prep time: 10 minutes I **Cooking time:** 40 minutes I
Servings: 4

Ingredients:

- 1 yellow onion, chopped
- 4 pork chops
- 2 tablespoons olive oil
- 1 tablespoon sweet paprika
- 2 tablespoons balsamic vinegar
- ¼ cup kalamata olives, pitted and chopped
- 1 tablespoon cilantro, chopped
- A pinch of sea salt and black pepper

Directions:

1. Heat up a pan with the oil over medium heat, add the onion and sauté for 5 minutes.
2. Add the meat and brown for 5 minutes more.
3. Add the rest of the ingredients, toss, cook over medium heat for 30 minutes, divide between plates and serve.

Nutrition info per serving: calories 280, fat 11, fiber 6, carbs 10, protein 21

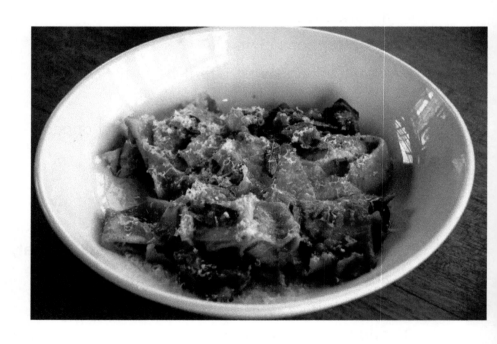

Pork and Salsa

Prep time: 10 minutes I **Cooking time:** 15 minutes I

Servings: 4

Ingredients:

- 4 pork chops
- 1 tablespoon olive oil
- 4 scallions, chopped
- 1 teaspoon cumin, ground
- ½ tablespoon hot paprika
- 1 teaspoon garlic powder
- A pinch of sea salt and black pepper
- 1 small red onion, chopped
- 2 tomatoes, cubed
- 2 tablespoons lime juice
- 1 jalapeno, chopped
- ¼ cup cilantro, chopped
- 1 tablespoon lime juice

Directions:

1. Heat up a pan with the oil over medium heat, add the scallions and sauté for 5 minutes.

2. Add the meat, cumin paprika, garlic powder, salt and pepper, toss, cook for 5 minutes on each side and divide between plates.
3. In a bowl, combine the tomatoes with the remaining ingredients, toss, divide next to the pork chops and serve.

Nutrition info per serving: calories 313, fat 23.7, fiber 1.7, carbs 5.9, protein 19.2

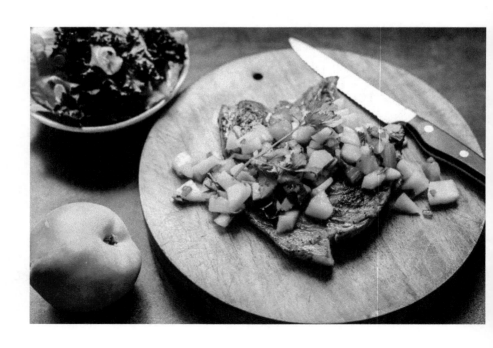

Rosemary Pork and Shallots Mix

Prep time: 10 minutes I **Cooking time:** 35 minutes I
Servings: 4

Ingredients:

- 2 shallots, chopped
- 1 pound pork stew meat, cubed
- 2 garlic cloves, minced
- 2 tablespoons olive oil
- ¼ cup Dijon mustard
- 2 tablespoons chives, chopped
- 1 teaspoon cumin, ground
- 1 teaspoon rosemary, dried
- A pinch of sea salt and black pepper

Directions:

1. Heat up a pan with the oil over medium-high heat, add the shallots and sauté for 5 minutes.
2. Add the meat and brown for 5 minutes more.
3. Add the rest of the ingredients, toss, cook over medium heat for 25 minutes more.
4. Divide the mix between plates and serve.

Nutrition info per serving: calories 280, fat 14.3, fiber 6, carbs 11.8, protein 17

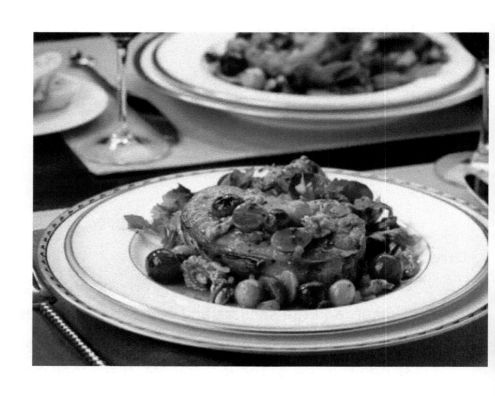

Pork with Tomatoes

Prep time: 10 minutes I **Cooking time:** 35 minutes I
Servings: 4

Ingredients:

- 2 tomatoes, cubed
- 2 pounds pork stew meat, cubed
- 4 scallions, chopped
- 2 tablespoons olive oil
- 1 zucchini, sliced
- Juice of 1 lime
- 2 tablespoons chili powder
- ½ tablespoons cumin powder
- A pinch of sea salt and black pepper

Directions:

1. Heat up a pan with the oil over medium heat, add the scallions and sauté for 5 minutes.
2. Add the meat and brown for 5 minutes more.
3. Add the tomatoes and the other ingredients, toss, cook over medium heat for 25 minutes more, divide between plates and serve.

Nutrition info per serving: calories 300, fat 5, fiber 2, carbs 12, protein 14

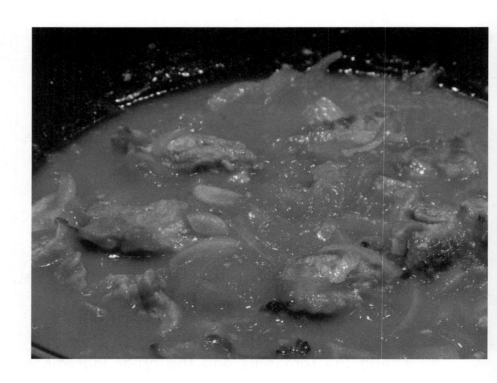

Pork and Sweet Potatoes

Prep time: 10 minutes I **Cooking time:** 35 minutes I
Servings: 4

Ingredients:

- 2 sweet potatoes, peeled and cut into wedges
- 4 pork chops
- 3 spring onions, chopped
- 1 tablespoon thyme, chopped
- 2 tablespoons olive oil
- 4 garlic cloves, minced
- A pinch of sea salt and black pepper
- ½ cup vegetable stock
- ½ tablespoon chives, chopped

Directions:

1. In a roasting pan, combine the pork chops with the potatoes and the other ingredients, toss gently and cook at 390 degrees F for 35 minutes.
2. Divide everything between plates and serve.

Nutrition info per serving: calories 210, fat 12.2, fiber 5.2, carbs 12, protein 10

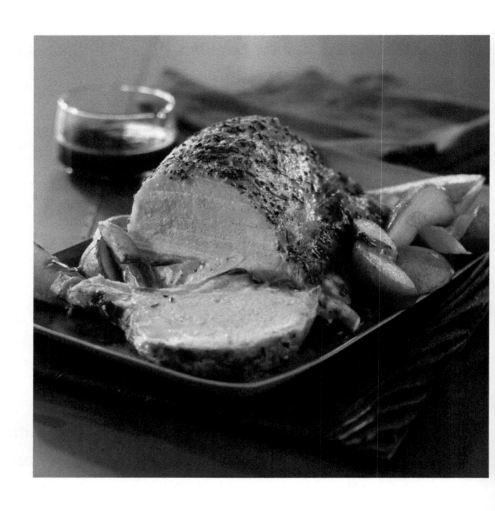

Pork with Pears

Prep time: 10 minutes I **Cooking time:** 35 minutes I

Servings: 4

Ingredients:

- 2 green onions, chopped
- 2 tablespoons avocado oil
- 2 pounds pork roast, sliced
- ½ cup coconut aminos
- 1 tablespoon ginger, minced
- 2 pears, cored and cut into wedges
- ¼ cup vegetable stock
- 1 tablespoon chives, chopped

Directions:

1. Heat up a pan with the oil over medium heat, add the onions and the meat and brown for 2 minutes on each side.
2. Add the rest of the ingredients, toss gently and bake at 390 degrees F for 30 minutes.
3. Divide the mix between plates and serve.

Nutrition info per serving: calories 220, fat 13.3, fiber 2, carbs 16.5, protein 8

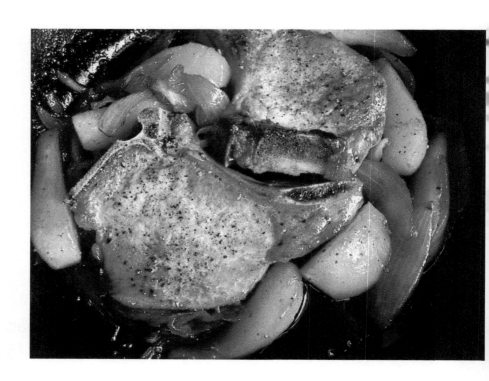

Turmeric Pork and Artichokes

Prep time: 10 minutes I **Cooking time:** 35 minutes I
Servings: 4

Ingredients:

- 2 tablespoons balsamic vinegar
- 1 cup artichoke hearts, quartered
- 2 tablespoons olive oil
- 2 pounds pork stew meat, cubed
- 2 tablespoons parsley, chopped
- 1 teaspoon cumin, ground
- 1 teaspoon turmeric powder
- 2 garlic cloves, minced
- A pinch of sea salt and black pepper

Directions:

1. Heat up a pan with the oil over medium heat, add the meat and brown for 5 minutes.
2. Add the artichokes, the vinegar and the other ingredients, toss, cook over medium heat for 30 minutes, divide between plates and serve.

Nutrition info per serving: calories 260, fat 5, fiber 4, carbs 11, protein 20

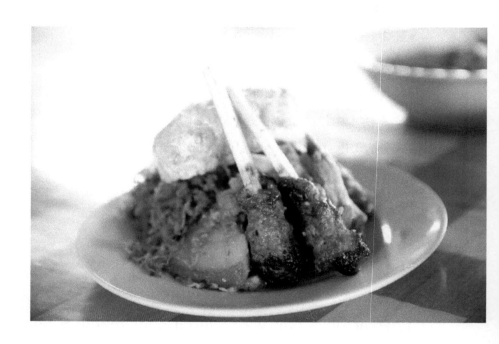

Pork with Lime Mushrooms Mix

Prep time: 10 minutes I **Cooking time:** 25 minutes I
Servings: 4

Ingredients:

- 2 tablespoons olive oil
- ½ teaspoon oregano, dried
- 4 pork chops
- 2 garlic cloves, minced
- Juice of 1 lime
- ¼ cup cilantro, chopped
- A pinch of sea salt and black pepper
- 1 cup white mushrooms, halved
- 2 tablespoons balsamic vinegar

Directions:

1. Heat up a pan with the oil over medium heat, add the pork chops and brown for 2 minutes on each side.
2. Add the rest of the ingredients, toss, cook over medium heat for 20 minutes, divide between plates and serve.

Nutrition info per serving: calories 220, fat 6, fiber 8, carbs 14.2, protein 20

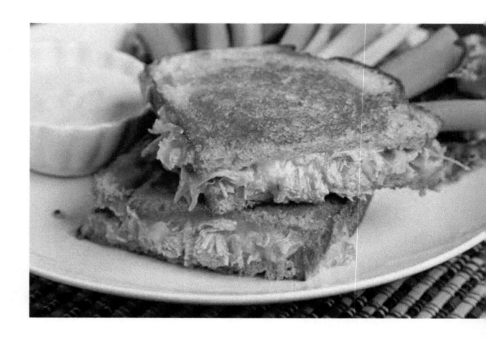

Oregano Hot Pork

Prep time: 10 minutes I **Cooking time:** 8 hours I
Servings: 4

Ingredients:

- 2 pounds pork roast, sliced
- 2 tablespoons oregano, chopped
- ¼ cup balsamic vinegar
- 1 cup tomato paste
- 1 tablespoon sweet paprika
- 1 teaspoon onion powder
- 2 tablespoons chili powder
- 2 garlic cloves, minced
- A pinch of salt and black pepper

Directions:

1. In your slow cooker, combine the roast with the oregano, the vinegar and the other ingredients, toss, put the lid on and cook on Low for 8 hours.
2. Divide everything between plates and serve.

Nutrition info per serving: calories 300, fat 5, fiber 2, carbs 12, protein 24

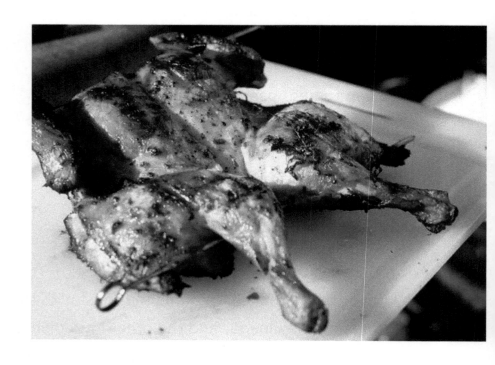

Creamy Pork

Prep time: 10 minutes I **Cooking time:** 35 minutes I
Servings: 4

Ingredients:

- 2 pounds pork stew meat, cubed
- 2 tablespoons avocado oil
- 1 cup tomatoes, cubed
- 1 cup coconut cream
- 1 tablespoon mint, chopped
- 1 jalapeno pepper, chopped
- A pinch of sea salt and black pepper
- 1 tablespoons hot pepper
- 2 tablespoons lemon juice

Directions:

1. Heat up a pan with the oil over medium heat, add the meat and brown for 5 minutes.
2. Add the rest of the ingredients, toss, cook over medium heat for 30 minutes more, divide between plates and serve.

Nutrition info per serving: calories 230, fat 4, fiber 6, carbs 9, protein 14

Pork and Onion Sauce

Prep time: 10 minutes I **Cooking time:** 35 minutes I
Servings: 4

Ingredients:

- 1 yellow onion, chopped
- 4 scallions, chopped
- 2 tablespoons avocado oil
- 1 tablespoon rosemary, chopped
- 1 tablespoon lemon zest, grated
- 2 pounds pork roast, sliced
- 2 tablespoons balsamic vinegar
- ½ cup vegetable stock
- A pinch of sea salt and black pepper

Directions:

1. Heat up a pan with the oil over medium heat, add the onion and the scallions and sauté for 5 minutes.
2. Add the rest of the ingredients except the meat, stir, and simmer for 5 minutes.
3. Add the meat, toss gently, cook over medium heat for 25 minutes, divide between plates and serve.

Nutrition info per serving: calories 217, fat 11, fiber 1, carbs 6, protein 14

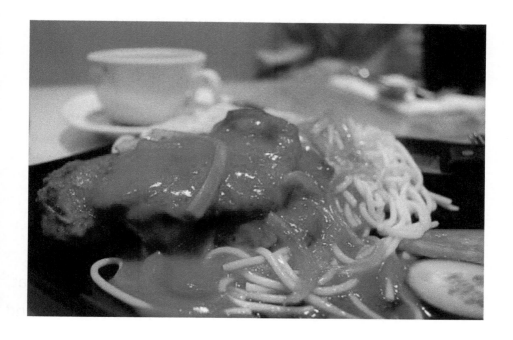

Ground Pork and Veggies Pan

Prep time: 5 minutes I **Cooking time:** 15 minutes I **Servings:** 4

Ingredients:

- 2 garlic cloves, minced
- 2 red chilies, chopped
- 2 tablespoons olive oil
- 2 pounds pork stew meat, ground
- 1 red bell pepper, chopped
- 1 green bell pepper, chopped
- 1 tomato, cubed
- ½ cup mushrooms, halved
- A pinch of sea salt and black pepper
- 1 tablespoon basil, chopped
- 2 tablespoons coconut aminos

Directions:

1. Heat up a pan with the oil over medium heat, add the garlic, chilies, bell peppers, tomato and the mushrooms and sauté for 5 minutes.
2. Add the meat and the rest of the ingredients, toss, cook over medium heat for 10 minutes more, divide between plates and serve.

Nutrition info per serving: calories 200, fat 3, fiber 5, carbs 7, protein 17

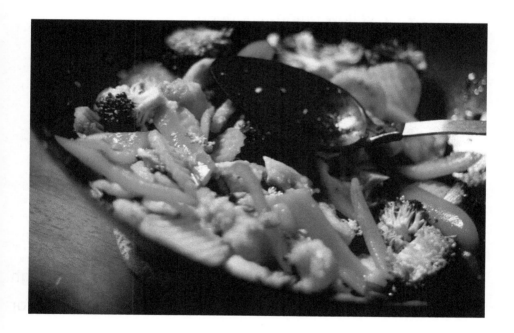

Pork and Squash

Prep time: 10 minutes I **Cooking time:** 35 minutes I
Servings: 4

Ingredients:

- 1 pound pork stew meat, cubed
- 1 butternut squash, peeled and cubed
- 1 yellow onion, chopped
- 2 tablespoons olive oil
- 2 garlic cloves, minced
- ½ teaspoon garam masala
- ½ teaspoon nutmeg, ground
- 1 teaspoon chili flakes, crushed
- 1 tablespoon balsamic vinegar
- A pinch of sea salt and black pepper

Directions:

1. Heat up a pan with the oil over medium-high heat, add the onion and the garlic and sauté for 5 minutes.
2. Add the meat and brown for another 5 minutes.
3. Add the rest of the ingredients, toss, cook over medium heat for 25 minutes, divide between plates and serve.

Nutrition info per serving: calories 348, fat 18.2, fiber 2.1, carbs 11.4, protein 34.3

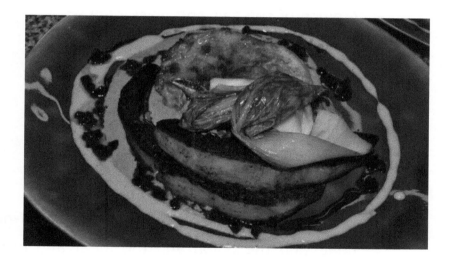

Pork with Greens

Prep time: 10 minutes I **Cooking time:** 35 minutes I
Servings: 4

Ingredients:

- 1 pound pork stew meat, cut into strips
- 2 tablespoons olive oil
- 1 yellow onion, chopped
- A pinch of sea salt and black pepper
- 1 cup green cabbage, shredded
- ½ cup baby kale
- 2 tablespoons oregano, dried
- 2 tablespoons balsamic vinegar
- ¼ cup vegetable stock

Directions:

1. Heat up a pan with the oil over medium-high heat, add the onion and the meat and brown for 5 minutes.
2. Add the cabbage and the other ingredients, toss gently and bake everything at 390 degrees F for 30 minutes.
3. Divide the whole mix between plates and serve.

Nutrition info per serving: calories 331, fat 18.7, fiber 2.1, carbs 6.5, protein 34.2

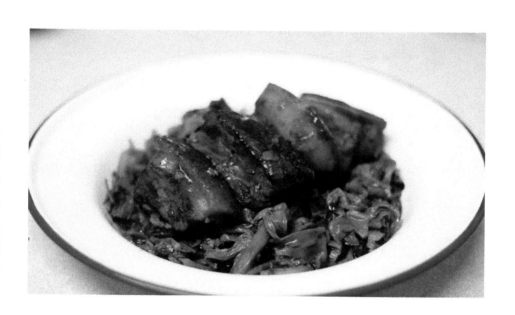

Pork and Cucumber Salad

Prep time: 5 minutes I **Cooking time:** 10 minutes I
Servings: 4

Ingredients:

- 1 pound pork stew meat, cut into strips
- 3 tablespoons olive oil
- 4 scallions, chopped
- 2 tablespoons lemon juice
- 2 tablespoons balsamic vinegar
- 2 cups mixed salad greens
- 1 avocado, peeled, pitted and roughly cubed
- 1 cucumber, sliced
- 2 tomatoes, cubed
- A pinch of salt and black pepper

Directions:

1. Heat up a pan with 2 tablespoons of oil over medium heat, add the scallions, the meat and the lemon juice, toss and cook for 10 minutes.
2. In a salad bowl, combine the salad greens with the meat and the remaining ingredients, toss and serve.

Nutrition info per serving: calories 225, fat 6.4, fiber 4, carbs 8, protein 11

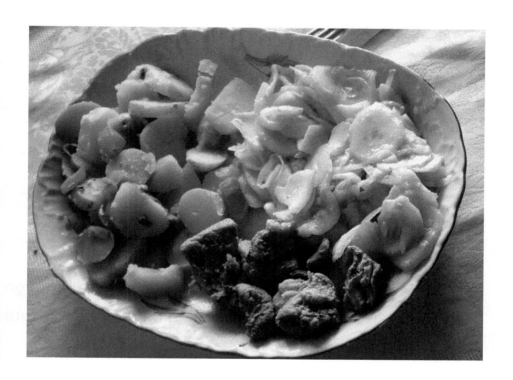

Pork Curry

Ingredients:

- 2 tablespoon olive oil
- 4 scallions, chopped
- 2 garlic cloves, minced
- 2 pounds pork stew meat, cubed
- 2 tablespoons red curry paste
- 1 teaspoon chili paste
- 2 tablespoons balsamic vinegar
- ¼ cup vegetable stock
- ¼ cup parsley, chopped

Directions:

1. Heat up a pan with the oil over medium-high heat, add the scallions and the garlic and sauté for 5 minutes.
2. Add the meat and brown for 5 minutes more.
3. Add the remaining ingredients, toss, cook over medium heat for 20 minutes, divide between plates and serve.

Nutrition info per serving: calories 220, fat 3, fiber 4, carbs 7, protein 12

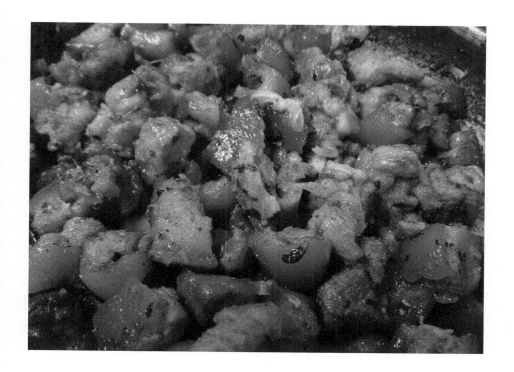

Italian Roast

Ingredients:

- 2 pounds pork roast
- 3 tablespoons olive oil
- 2 teaspoons oregano, dried
- 1 tablespoon Italian seasoning
- 1 teaspoon rosemary, dried
- 1 teaspoon basil, dried
- 3 garlic cloves, minced
- ¼ cup vegetable stock
- A pinch of salt and black pepper

Directions:

1. In a baking pan, combine the pork roast with the oil, the oregano and the other ingredients, toss and bake at 390 degrees F for 1 hour.
2. Slice the roast, divide it and the other ingredients between plates and serve.

Nutrition info per serving: calories 580, fat 33.6, fiber 0.5, carbs 2.3, protein 64.9

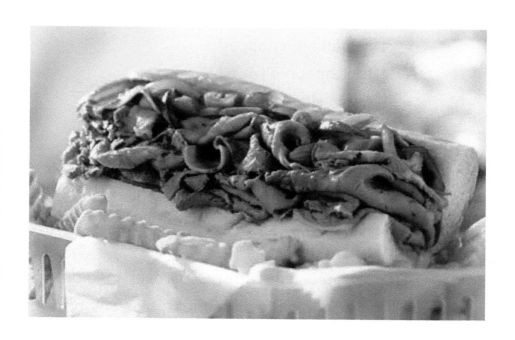

Chives Pork Mix

Prep time: 10 minutes I **Cooking time:** 45 minutes I
Servings: 8

Ingredients:

- 2 pounds pork meat, boneless and cubed
- 1 red onion, chopped
- 1 tablespoon olive oil
- 3 garlic cloves, minced
- 1 cup beef stock
- 2 tablespoons sweet paprika
- Black pepper to the taste
- 1 tablespoon chives, chopped

Directions:

1. Heat up a pan with the oil over medium heat, add the onion and the meat, toss and brown for 5 minutes.
2. Add the rest of the ingredients, toss, reduce heat to medium, cover and cook for 40 minutes.
3. Divide the mix between plates and serve.

Nutrition info per serving: calories 407, fat 35.4, fiber 1, carbs 5, protein 14.9

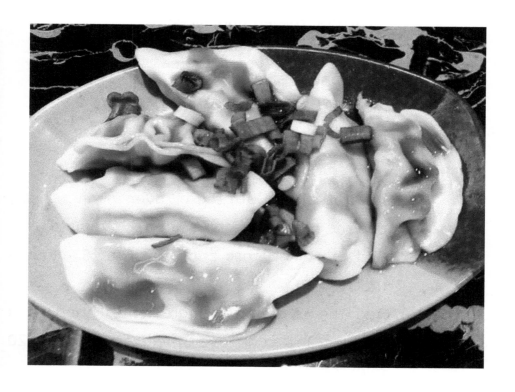

Pork with Carrots

Prep time: 10 minutes I **Cooking time:** 30 minutes I **Servings:** 4

Ingredients:

- 1 pound pork stew meat, cubed
- ¼ cup veggie stock
- 2 carrots, peeled and sliced
- 2 tablespoons olive oil
- 1 red onion, sliced
- 2 teaspoons sweet paprika
- Black pepper to the taste

Directions:

1. Heat up a pan with the oil over medium heat, add the onion, stir and sauté for 5 minutes.
2. Add the meat, toss and brown for 5 minutes more.
3. Add the rest of the ingredients, bring to a simmer and cook over medium heat for 20 minutes.
4. Divide the mix between plates and serve.

Nutrition info per serving: calories 328, fat 18.1, fiber 1.8, carbs 6.4, protein 34

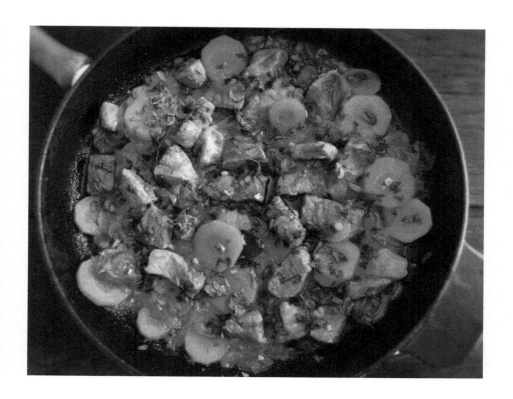

Ginger Pork

Prep time: 10 minutes I **Cooking time:** 35 minutes I
Servings: 4

Ingredients:

- 2 red onions, sliced
- 2 green onions, chopped
- 1 tablespoon olive oil
- 2 teaspoons ginger, grated
- 4 pork chops
- 3 garlic cloves, chopped
- Black pepper to the taste
- 1 carrot, chopped
- 1 cup beef stock
- 2 tablespoons tomato paste
- 1 tablespoon cilantro, chopped

Directions:

1. Heat up a pan with the oil over medium heat, add the green and red onions, toss and sauté them for 3 minutes.
2. Add the garlic and the ginger, toss and cook for 2 minutes more.
3. Add the pork chops and cook them for 2 minutes on each side.
4. Add the rest of the ingredients, bring to a simmer and cook over medium heat for 25 minutes more.
5. Divide the mix between plates and serve.

Nutrition info per serving: calories 332, fat 23.6, fiber 2.3, carbs 10.1, protein 19.9

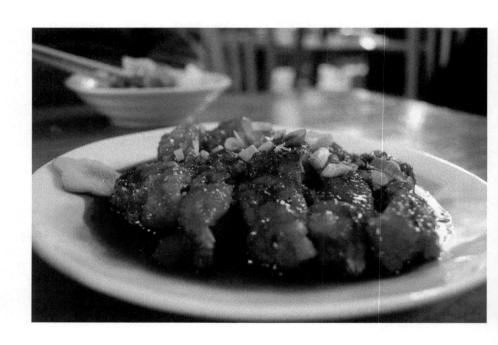

Pork and Cherry Tomatoes

Prep time: 10 minutes I **Cooking time:** 45 minutes I
Servings: 4

Ingredients:

- ½ cup beef stock
- 2 tablespoons olive oil
- 2 pounds pork stew meat, cubed
- 1 teaspoon coriander, ground
- 2 teaspoons cumin, ground
- Black pepper to the taste
- 1 cup cherry tomatoes, halved
- 4 garlic cloves, minced
- 1 tablespoon cilantro, chopped

Directions:

1. Heat up a pan with the oil over medium heat, add the garlic and the meat, toss and brown for 5 minutes.
2. Add the stock and the other ingredients, bring to a simmer and cook over medium heat for 40 minutes.
3. Divide everything between plates and serve.

Nutrition info per serving: calories 559, fat 29.3, fiber 0.7, carbs 3.2, protein 67.4

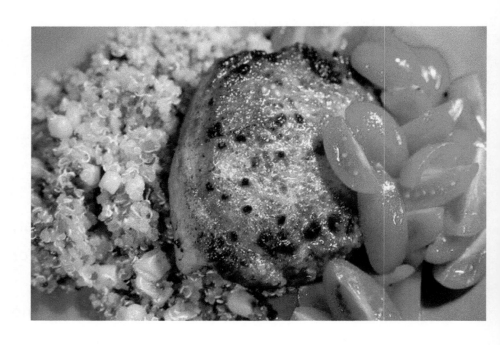

Pork Bowls

Prep time: 10 minutes I **Cooking time:** 20 minutes I
Servings: 4

Ingredients:

- 2 tablespoons balsamic vinegar
- 1/3 cup coconut aminos
- 1 tablespoon olive oil
- 4 ounces mixed salad greens
- 1 cup cherry tomatoes, halved
- 4 ounces pork stew meat, cut into strips
- 1 tablespoon chives, chopped

Directions:

1. Heat up a pan with the oil over medium heat, add the pork, aminos and the vinegar, toss and cook for 15 minutes.
2. Add the salad greens and the other ingredients, toss, cook for 5 minutes more, divide into bowls and serve.

Nutrition info per serving: calories 125, fat 6.4, fiber 0.6, carbs 6.8, protein 9.1

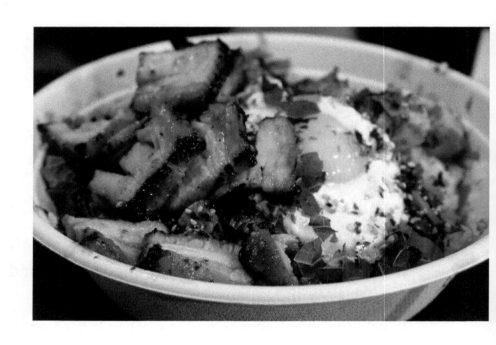

Pork and Tomato Passata Pan

Prep time: 10 minutes I **Cooking time:** 25 minutes I
Servings: 4

Ingredients:

- 1 pound pork butt, trimmed and cubed
- 1 tablespoon olive oil
- 1 yellow onion, chopped
- 3 garlic cloves, minced
- 1 tablespoon thyme, dried
- 1 cup chicken stock
- 2 tablespoons tomato passata
- 1 tablespoon cilantro, chopped

Directions:

1. Heat up a pan with the oil over medium-high heat, add the onion and the garlic, toss and cook for 5 minutes.
2. Add the meat, toss and cook for 5 more minutes.
3. Add the rest of the ingredients, toss, bring to a simmer, reduce heat to medium and cook the mix for 15 minutes more.

4. Divide the mix between plates and serve right away.

Nutrition info per serving: calories 281, fat 11.2, fiber 1.4, carbs 6.8, protein 37.1

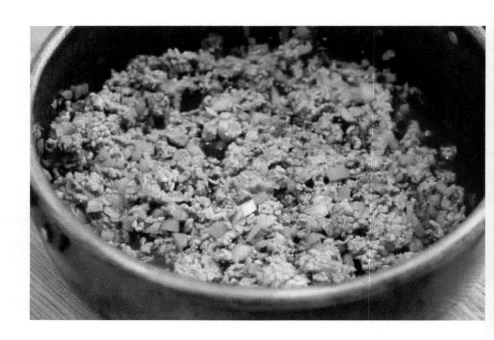

Marjoram Pork

Prep time: 10 minutes I **Cooking time:** 30 minutes I
Servings: 4

Ingredients:

- 2 pounds pork loin boneless, trimmed and cubed
- 2 tablespoons avocado oil
- ¾ cup veggie stock
- ½ tablespoon garlic powder
- 1 tablespoon marjoram, chopped
- 1 teaspoon sweet paprika
- Black pepper to the taste

Directions:

1. Heat up a pan with the oil over medium-high heat, add the meat, garlic powder and the marjoram, toss and cook for 10 minutes.
2. Add the other ingredients, toss, bring to a simmer, reduce heat to medium and cook the mix for 20 minutes more.
3. Divide everything between plates and serve.

Nutrition info per serving: calories 359, fat 9.1, fiber 2.1, carbs 5.7, protein 61.4

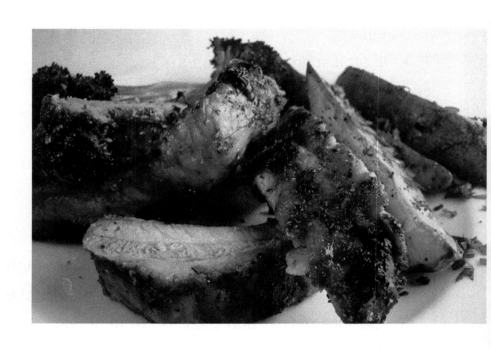

Nutmeg Pork

Prep time: 10 minutes I **Cooking time:** 8 hours I
0Servings: 4

Ingredients:

- 3 tablespoons olive oil
- 2 pounds pork shoulder roast
- 2 teaspoons sweet paprika
- 1 teaspoon garlic powder
- 1 teaspoon onion powder
- 1 teaspoon nutmeg, ground
- 1 teaspoon allspice, ground
- Black pepper to the taste
- 1 cup veggie stock

Directions:

1. In your slow cooker, combine the roast with the oil and the other ingredients, toss, put the lid on and cook on Low for 8 hours.
2. Slice the roast, divide it between plates and serve with the cooking juices drizzled on top.

Nutrition info per serving: calories 689, fat 57.1, fiber 1, carbs 3.2, protein 38.8

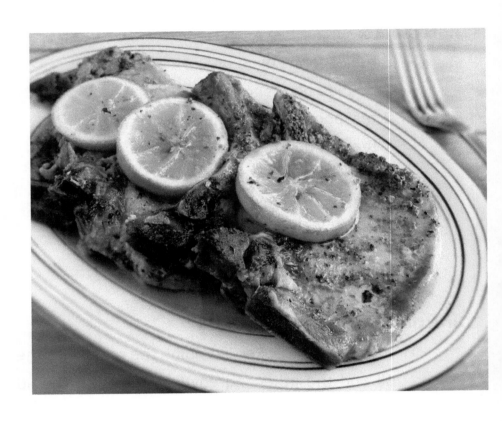

Chives Pork and Celery

Prep time: 10 minutes I **Cooking time:** 35 minutes I
Servings: 4

Ingredients:

- 2 pounds pork stew meat, cubed
- 2 tablespoons olive oil
- 1 cup veggie stock
- 1 celery stalk, chopped
- 1 teaspoon black peppercorns
- 2 shallots, chopped
- 1 tablespoon chives, chopped
- 1 cup coconut cream
- Black pepper to the taste

Directions:

1. Heat up a pan with the oil over medium heat, add the shallots and the meat, toss and brown for 5 minutes.
2. Add the celery and the other ingredients, toss, bring to a simmer and cook over medium heat for 30 minutes more.
3. Divide everything between plates and serve right away.

Nutrition info per serving: calories 690, fat 43.3, fiber 1.8, carbs 5.7, protein 6.2

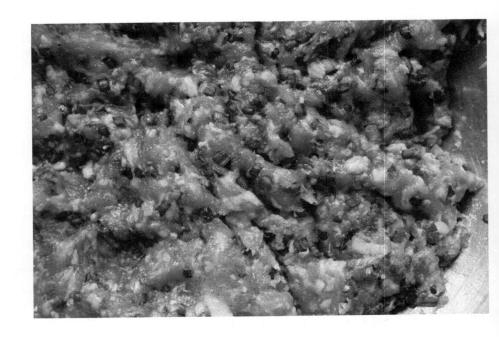

Pork and Red Onion Mix

Prep time: 10 minutes I **Cooking time:** 30 minutes I
Servings: 4

Ingredients:

- 2 garlic cloves, minced
- 2 pounds pork stew meat, ground
- 2 cups cherry tomatoes, halved
- 1 tablespoon olive oil
- Black pepper to the taste
- 1 red onion, chopped
- ½ cup veggie stock
- 2 tablespoons tomato passata
- 1 tablespoon parsley, chopped

Directions:

1. Heat up a pan with the oil over medium heat, add the onion and the garlic, toss and sauté for 5 minutes.
2. Add the meat and brown it for 5 minutes more.
3. Add the rest of the ingredients, toss, bring to a simmer, cook over medium heat for 20 minutes more, divide into bowls and serve.

Nutrition info per serving: calories 558, fat 25.6, fiber 2.4, carbs 10.1, protein 68.7

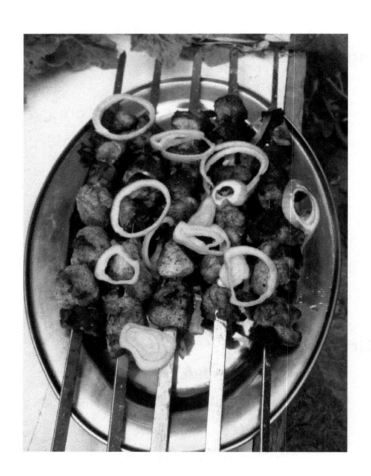

Pork Chops and Artichokes

Prep time: 10 minutes I **Cooking time:** 35 minutes I
Servings: 4

Ingredients:

- 4 pork chops
- 1 cup artichoke hearts, halved
- 2 tablespoons olive oil
- 1 teaspoon smoked paprika
- 1 tablespoon sage, chopped
- 2 garlic cloves, minced
- 1 tablespoon lemon juice
- Black pepper to the taste

Directions:

1. In a baking dish, combine the pork chops with the oil and the other ingredients, toss, introduce in the oven and bake at 400 degrees F for 35 minutes.
2. Divide the pork chops between plates and serve with a side salad.

Nutrition info per serving: calories 263, fat 12.4, fiber 6, carbs 22.2, protein 16

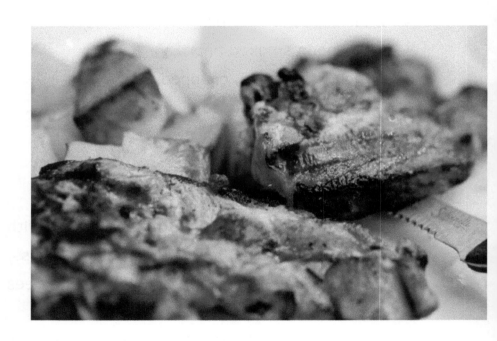

Pork and Eggplant

Prep time: 10 minutes I **Cooking time:** 30 minutes I
Servings: 4

Ingredients:

- 1 pound pork stew meat, cubed
- 1 eggplant, cubed
- 1 tablespoon coconut aminos
- 1 teaspoon five spice
- 2 garlic cloves, minced
- 2 Thai chilies, chopped
- 2 tablespoons olive oil
- 2 tablespoons tomato passata
- 1 tablespoon cilantro, chopped
- ½ cup veggie stock

Directions:

1. Heat up a pan with the oil over medium-high heat, add the garlic, chilies and the meat and brown for 6 minutes.
2. Add the eggplant and the other ingredients, bring to a simmer and cook over medium heat for 24 minutes.
3. Divide the mix between plates and serve.

Nutrition info per serving: calories 320, fat 13.4, fiber 5.2, carbs 22.8, protein 14

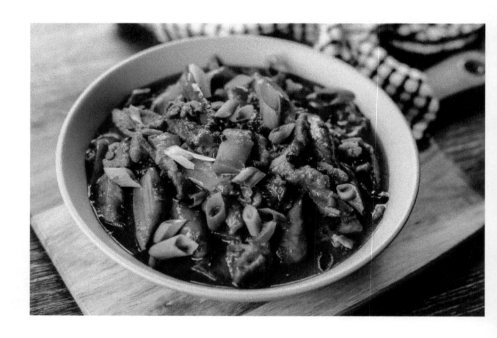

Pork and Lime Scallions

Prep time: 10 minutes I **Cooking time:** 30 minutes I
Servings: 4

Ingredients:

- 2 tablespoons lime juice
- 4 scallions, chopped
- 1 pound pork stew meat, cubed
- 2 garlic cloves, minced
- 2 tablespoons olive oil
- Black pepper to the taste
- ½ cup veggie stock
- 1 tablespoon cilantro, chopped

Directions:

1. Heat up a pan with the oil over medium heat, add the scallions and the garlic, toss and cook for 5 minutes.
2. Add the meat, toss and cook for 5 minutes more.
3. Add the rest of the ingredients, bring to a simmer and cook over medium heat for 20 minutes.
4. Divide the mix between plates and serve.

Nutrition info per serving: calories 273, fat 22.4, fiber 5, carbs 12.5, protein 18

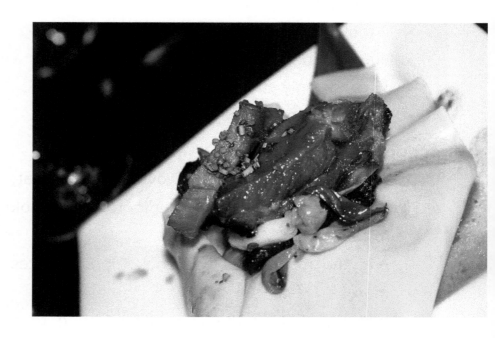

Balsamic Coriander Pork

Prep time: 10 minutes I **Cooking time:** 30 minutes I
Servings: 4

Ingredients:

- 1 red onion, sliced
- 1 pound pork stew meat, cubed
- 2 red chilies, chopped
- 2 tablespoons balsamic vinegar
- ½ cup coriander leaves, chopped
- Black pepper to the taste
- 2 tablespoons olive oil
- 1 tablespoon tomato sauce

Directions:

1. Heat up a pan with the oil over medium heat, add the onion and the chilies, toss and cook for 5 minutes.
2. Add the meat, toss and cook for 5 minutes more.
3. Add the rest of the ingredients, toss, bring to a simmer and cook over medium heat for 20 minutes more.
4. Divide everything between plates and serve right away.

Nutrition info per serving: calories 331, fat 13.3, fiber 5, carbs 22.7, protein 17

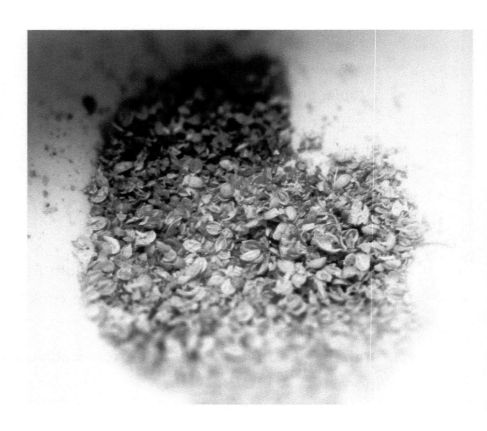

Pesto Pork Chops

Prep time: 10 minutes I **Cooking time:** 36 minutes I
Servings: 4

Ingredients:

- 2 tablespoons olive oil
- 2 spring onions, chopped
- 1 pound pork chops
- 2 tablespoons basil pesto
- 1 cup cherry tomatoes, cubed
- 2 tablespoons tomato passata
- ½ cup parsley, chopped
- ½ cup veggie stock
- Black pepper to the taste

Directions:

1. Heat up a pan with the olive oil over medium-high heat, add the spring onions and the pork chops, and brown for 3 minutes on each side.
2. Add the pesto and the other ingredients, toss gently, bring to a simmer and cook over medium heat for 30 minutes more.
3. Divide everything between plates and serve.

Nutrition info per serving: calories 293, fat 11.3, fiber 4.2, carbs 22.2, protein 14

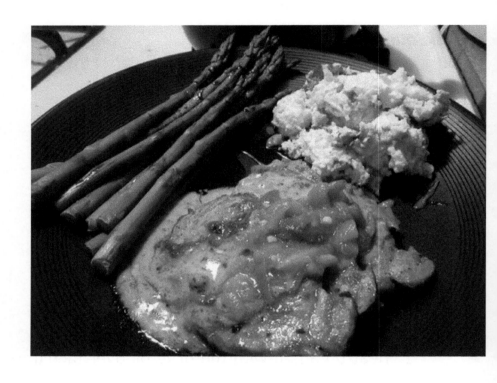

Pork and Mixed Peppers

Prep time: 10 minutes I **Cooking time:** 1 hour I
Servings: 4

Ingredients:

- 1 green bell pepper, chopped
- 1 red bell pepper, chopped
- 1 yellow bell pepper, chopped
- 1 red onion, chopped
- 1 pound pork chops
- 1 tablespoon olive oil
- Black pepper to the taste
- 26 ounces tomatoes, chopped
- 2 tablespoons parsley, chopped

Directions:

1. Grease a roasting pan with the oil, arrange the pork chops inside and add the other ingredients on top.
2. Bake at 390 degrees F for 1 hour, divide everything between plates and serve.

Nutrition info per serving: calories 284, fat 11.6, fiber 2.6, carbs 22.2, protein 14

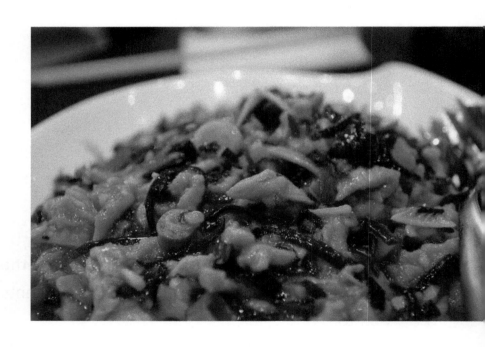

Cumin Chili Lamb Mix

Prep time: 10 minutes I **Cooking time:** 25 minutes I
Servings: 4

Ingredients:

- 1 tablespoon olive oil
- 1 red onion, chopped
- 1 cup cherry tomatoes, halved
- 1 pound lamb stew meat, ground
- 1 tablespoon chili powder
- Black pepper to the taste
- 2 teaspoons cumin, ground
- 1 cup veggie stock
- 2 tablespoons cilantro, chopped

Directions:

1. Heat up the a pan with the oil over medium-high heat, add the onion, lamb and chili powder, toss and cook for 10 minutes.
2. Add the rest of the ingredients, toss, cook over medium heat for 15 minutes more.
3. Divide into bowls and serve.

Nutrition info per serving: calories 320, fat 12,7, fiber 6, carbs 14.3, protein 22

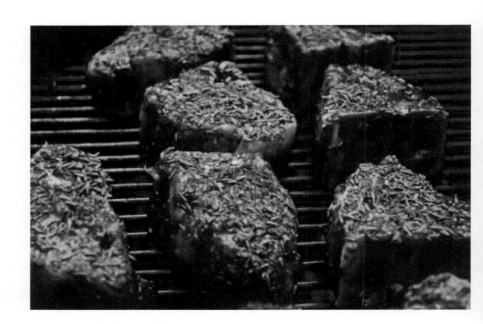

Beef with Radishes

Prep time: 10 minutes I **Cooking time:** 35 minutes I
Servings: 4

Ingredients:

- 1 pound beef stew meat, cubed
- 1 cup radishes, cubed
- ½ pound green beans, trimmed and halved
- 1 yellow onion, chopped
- 1 tablespoon olive oil
- 2 garlic cloves, minced
- 1 cup tomatoes, chopped
- 2 teaspoons oregano, dried
- Black pepper to the taste

Directions:

1. Heat up a pan with the oil over medium-high heat, add the onion and the garlic, toss and cook for 5 minutes.
2. Add the meat, toss and cook for 5 minutes more.
3. Add the rest of the ingredients, bring to a simmer and cook over medium heat for 25 minutes.
4. Divide everything into bowls and serve.

Nutrition info per serving: calories 289, fat 12, fiber 8, carbs 13.2, protein 20

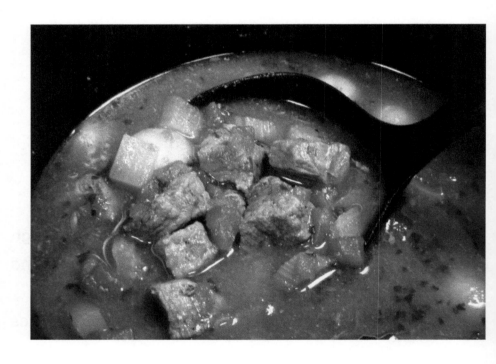

Lamb and Mushrooms

Prep time: 10 minutes I **Cooking time:** 40 minutes I
Servings: 4

Ingredients:

- 1 pound lamb shoulder, boneless and cubed
- 8 white mushrooms, halved
- 2 tablespoons olive oil
- 1 yellow onion, chopped
- 2 garlic cloves, minced
- 1 an ½ tablespoons fennel powder
- Black pepper to the taste
- A bunch of scallions, chopped
- 1 cup veggie stock

Directions:

1. Heat up a pan with the oil over medium heat, add the onion and the garlic, toss and cook for 5 minutes.
2. Add the meat and the mushrooms, toss and cook for 5 minutes more.
3. Add the other ingredients, toss, bring to a simmer and cook over medium heat for 30 minutes.
4. Divide the mix into bowls and serve.

Nutrition info per serving: calories 290, fat 15.3, fiber 7, carbs 14.9, protein 14

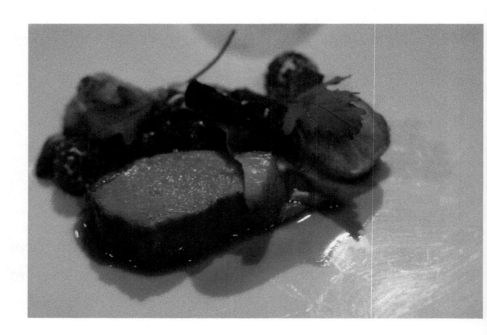

Beef and Spinach

Prep time: 10 minutes I **Cooking time:** 30 minutes I
Servings: 4

Ingredients:

- 1 pound beef, ground
- 2 tablespoons olive oil
- 1 red onion, chopped
- ½ pound baby spinach
- 4 garlic cloves, minced
- ½ cup veggie stock
- ½ cup tomatoes, chopped
- Black pepper to the taste
- 1 tablespoon chives, chopped

Directions:

1. Heat up a pan with the oil over medium-high heat, add the onion and the garlic, toss and cook for 5 minutes.
2. Add the meat, toss and brown for 5 minutes more.
3. Add the rest of the ingredients except the spinach, toss, bring to a simmer, reduce heat to medium and cook for 15 minutes.

4. Add the spinach, toss, cook the mix for another 5 minutes, divide everything into bowls and serve.

Nutrition info per serving: calories 270, fat 12, fiber 6, carbs 22.2, protein 23

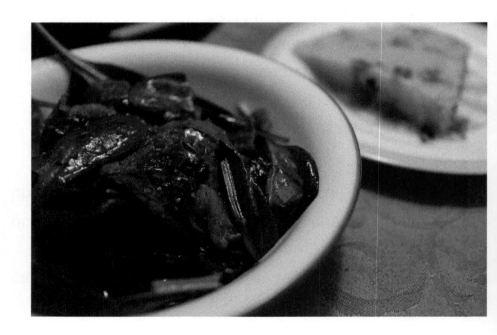

Pork with Tomatoes and Avocados

Prep time: 10 minutes I **Cooking time:** 15 minutes I
Servings: 4

Ingredients:

- 2 cups baby spinach
- 1 pound pork steak, cut into strips
- 1 tablespoon olive oil
- 1 cup cherry tomatoes, halved
- 2 avocados, peeled, pitted and cut into wedges
- 1 tablespoon balsamic vinegar
- ½ cup veggie stock

Directions:

1. Heat up a pan with the oil over medium-high heat, add the meat, toss and cook for 10 minutes.
2. Add the spinach and the other ingredients, toss, cook for 5 minutes more, divide into bowls and serve.

Nutrition info per serving: calories 390, fat 12.5, fiber 4, carbs 16.8, protein 13.5

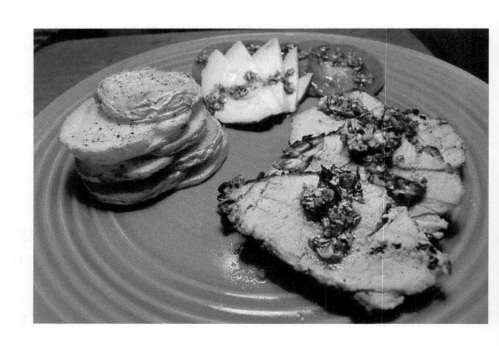

Pork with Apple Wedges

Prep time: 10 minutes I **Cooking time:** 40 minutes I
Servings: 4

Ingredients:

- 2 pounds pork stew meat, cut into strips
- 2 green apples, cored and cut into wedges
- 2 garlic cloves, minced
- 2 shallots, chopped
- 1 tablespoon sweet paprika
- ½ teaspoon chili powder
- 2 tablespoons avocado oil
- 1 cup chicken stock
- Black pepper to the taste
- A pinch of red chili pepper flakes

Directions:

1. Heat up a pan with the oil over medium heat,
   add the shallots and the garlic, toss and sauté
   for 5 minutes.
2. Add the meat and brown for another 5 minutes.

3. Add the apples and the other ingredients, toss, bring to a simmer and cook over medium heat for 30 minutes more.
4. Divide everything between plates and serve.

Nutrition info per serving: calories 365, fat 7, fiber 6, carbs 15.6, protein 32.4

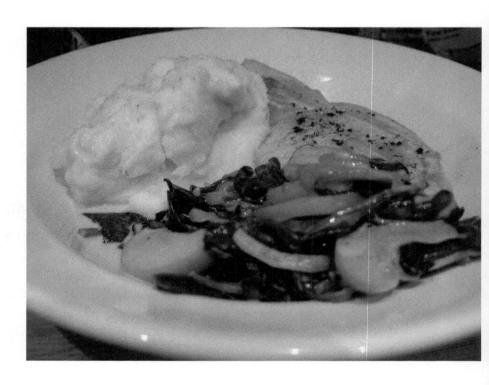

Tarragon Pork Chops

Prep time: 10 minutes

Cooking time: 1 hour and 10 minutes

Servings: 4

Ingredients:

- 4 pork chops
- 2 tablespoons olive oil
- 2 garlic cloves, minced
- ¼ cup veggie stock
- 1 tablespoon tarragon, chopped
- Black pepper to the taste
- 1 teaspoon chili powder
- ½ teaspoon onion powder

Directions:

1. In a roasting pan, combine the pork chops with the oil and the other ingredients, toss, introduce in the oven and bake at 390 degrees F for 1 hour and 10 minutes.
2. Divide the pork chops between plates and serve with a side salad.

Nutrition info per serving: calories 288, fat 5.5, fiber 6, carbs 12.7, protein 23

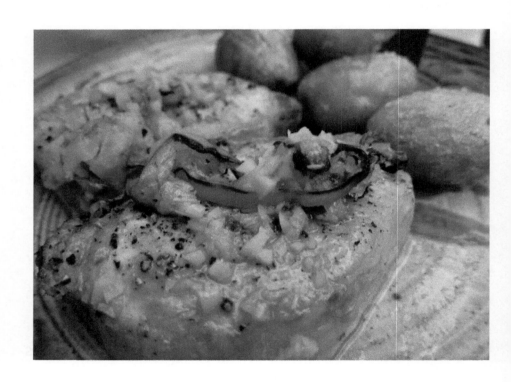

Coconut Pork Chops

Prep time: 10 minutes I **Cooking time:** 20 minutes I
Servings: 4

Ingredients:

- 2 tablespoons olive oil
- 4 pork chops
- 1 yellow onion, chopped
- 1 tablespoon chili powder
- 1 cup coconut milk
- ¼ cup cilantro, chopped

Directions:

1. Heat up a pan with the oil over medium-high heat, add the onion and the chili powder, toss and sauté for 5 minutes.
2. Add the pork chops and brown them for 2 minutes on each side.
3. Add the coconut milk, toss, bring to a simmer and cook over medium heat for 11 minutes more.
4. Add the cilantro, toss, divide everything into bowls and serve.

Nutrition info per serving: calories 310, fat 8, fiber 6, carbs 16.7, protein 22.1

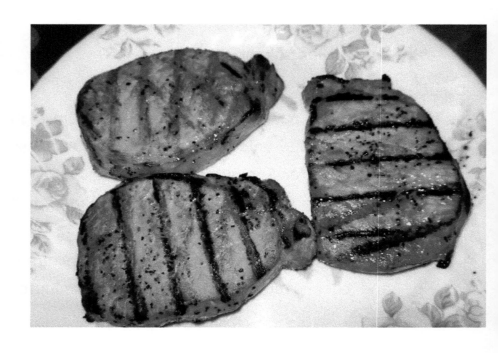

Pork with Peaches

Prep time: 10 minutes I **Cooking time:** 25 minutes I
Servings: 4

Ingredients:

- 2 pounds pork tenderloin, roughly cubed
- 2 peaches, stones removed and cut into quarters
- ¼ teaspoon onion powder
- 2 tablespoons olive oil
- ¼ teaspoon smoked paprika
- ¼ cup veggie stock
- Black pepper to the taste

Directions:

1. Heat up a pan with the oil over medium heat, add the meat, toss and cook for 10 minutes.
2. Add the peaches and the other ingredients, toss, bring to a simmer and cook over medium heat for 15 minutes more.
3. Divide the whole mix between plates and serve.

Nutrition info per serving: calories 290, fat 11.8, fiber 5.4, carbs 13.7, protein 24

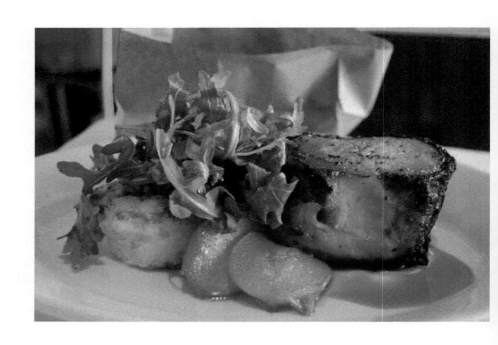

Lightning Source UK Ltd.
Milton Keynes UK
UKHW020802110621
385329UK00001B/122